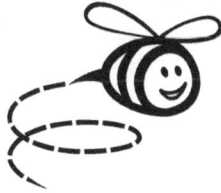

It's a Lot Like a
BEE STING

Things You Didn't Know About Childhood Cancer

SCOTT HETHERINGTON

Cover Illustration by
LINDA OBERLIN

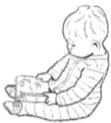

ISBN 978-0-9911382-1-0

Printed in the United States of America.

Preface

What Do I Know!?

A few weeks ago, a thought occurred to me while writing this. Why would someone want to read a book about me having cancer? I thought about it for a long time and realized that the answer to that question is the same reason I am writing this book in the first place! To give people hope. Hope that there is a finish line. That there is a reason to continue going to doctors' appointments and hospital stays; to continue chemotherapy, or radiation, or whatever treatment you are enduring.

I was 14 years old when I was diagnosed with leukemia. The entire time I was facing this illness, I always wanted to meet someone who had been through it, who had survived and now maybe had a life beyond needles and people in scrubs. Sometimes impossible tasks can seem more manageable when there is a goal in sight. We will assume that the main goal of anyone with any life threatening disease is to survive, but beyond that there needs to be something more concrete. Why do we want to survive? What is the reason? Those are the things that are the real end goals. This book is to show people who have or had cancer or who know someone with cancer, that there is a light at the end of the tunnel.

Now having said all of this, I am in no way a licensed physician or psychologist of any kind. My story is one that I hope can provide inspiration and support to anyone affected by the big 'C'.

Acknowledgements

To my mom, my dad, and my brother

Contents

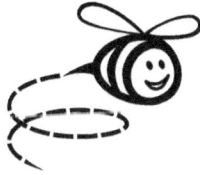

Chapter 1

I Won't Be Going to the Concert

WHEN I WAS fourteen, I was constantly making plans with friends at school and at home. My friends and I were, and still are, big concertgoers. We have seen a ton of bands. The acts we saw ranged from virtually unheard of bands like Jawbox and That Dog to huge bands like U2 and Smashing Pumpkins. When I was in the 9th grade, I had plans to go see a Weezer concert. This particular concert was special because it fell on a weeknight over the week of Spring Break in my freshman year of high school. Spring Break fell on the first week in April, and there would be no school the day after the show, nothing to do but sleep in late, watch TV, and play video games.

As the day of the show grew nearer, I was beginning to wonder if I was even going to be able to go. I had been missing school off and on for the better part of three weeks, dealing with nausea and fatigue. I wasn't sleeping well, and I had pain in my neck and head. These health problems started about a month earlier. At the beginning of March my mother, who was a travel agent at the time, surprised me by getting really cheap airfare to go to Paris, France. As a freshman I took an intro to French class and I had talked all year about how I would really like to go and see all of these things that we had been talking about in class all year. The trip was really great. My mom basically got us to Paris for about 4 days for just a few hundred dollars. We saw the Eiffel Tower, Notre Dame, the Louvre, all the big stuff. But this particular trip turned out to be very memorable in so many ways.

The morning we were scheduled to leave Paris, I woke up with paralysis in the left side of my face. I only had half a smile; I could only raise one eyebrow. Except for being in a foreign country and being scared out of my mind, I actually didn't feel bad. I wasn't in any pain, I didn't feel sick...I just had zero movement on the left side of my face. After a long plane ride back to the States, my dad met us at the gate and we all immediately went to the emergency room. It was a long night but it all amounted to the doctor telling me I had a severe ear infection, and the swelling in my ear canal pinched a nerve in my head that caused the paralysis. The condition is caused Bell's palsy and although I had never heard of it to that point, apparently quite a few people have it. I was told it could go away or I could have it for a long time. There was just no way of knowing. A long night had come to an end and it seemed as though the problem had been identified and mostly solved. My problem wasn't close to solved, though, and for the next few weeks my health didn't seem to be getting any better. I saw more and more doctors about my health. The more doctors I saw, the more tests they ran, and then they sent me to other doctors.

The final bell rang at school on Friday, March 31st. Spring Break had begun. I don't really remember the feeling because I didn't go to school that day. It was another day of feeling like crud. I had gone to see a neurologist about my face earlier in the week and he suggested they run some extensive blood tests. On that same Friday one of my blood tests came back a little abnormal. Apparently, I had an incredibly high white blood cell count. My mother drove me to the hospital to take another blood test. I remember riding in the car and telling my mom that this was going to be such a waste of time and that they were going to tell me that it wasn't a big deal. I have always wondered if my mom knew something that I didn't during that car ride. When we got to the hospital we waited in a tiny little white room for the results of the blood test. I remember that my dad was there, but I don't ever remember him showing up. Even more evidence that my mom knew something I didn't. She clearly called him and told him to meet us at the hospital. Not something she would do unless she knew something was up.

What seemed like hours later, the doctor came into my tiny little hospital waiting room, to tell me it was leukemia. The tiny little room at that moment seemed to get even smaller. After hearing the news I threw up. I didn't know it was possible to produce black vomit, but that night black vomit came out of my body. I mean I could understand if I had just eaten a pan of brownies, or maybe a bag of Hershey kisses. But with my nauseous state the previous few days, I had not eaten much of anything, much less something that would produce black vomit. Given the situation I think I handled the news fairly well.

After my vomiting a nurse came to run an IV, and I sat in that tiny little room with my mom and dad. The next few hours were much the same as a movie that you watch in fast forward, or those time delay documentaries that you watch on the Discovery Channel. I sat in slow motion while nurses, doctors, and orderlies came in and out at an extremely fast rate. Everything they did was to prep me for my extended stay at their hospital. After about an hour of a frenetic pace of people I didn't know, I was left with my parents alone to think about all of the things that had just fallen into my lap. I could tell my parents were scared, but they always did a good job of hiding their emotions around me. I guess it would have been a little unsettling to have your mother hysterical and screaming, "Oh shit you are going to die!" With a moment of silence I began to think about things that one thinks about when they are told they have cancer. I thought about my friends and school. What was I going to do about school? Then I thought about Spring Break and the concert. I guess I wasn't going to the concert? I realized that I needed to call my friend and share the news.

There was a phone in the little waiting room that could place outgoing calls. I dialed my friend and told him the news. There was silence on the other end. That happened a lot. At any moment there was the chaos of a hospital, the sounds, the lights, and then minutes later, silence. The phone call lasted just a few minutes. I told my friend to call the other guys and tell them the news if he could and that I would try to talk to him soon. After the call I sat thinking of what was to come. My parents and I exchanged a few small comments but for the most part it was a lot of thinking and more silence. Would I live? Would I die? Would it hurt? I had no idea what was to come. An hour later I was whisked away to my hospital room in whirlwind of noise, IV poles, and nurses. So much for silence.

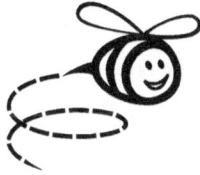

Chapter 2

The Pee Thermos

D URING MY STAY in the hospital, I had many visitors come to my hospital room. Mostly friends and family, but every now and again, someone would come to visit who I had never met. Visits are wonderful when you are in the hospital, but you are rarely looking your best. That is coupled with the fact that the hospital likes to run tests on *everything* that comes OUT of your body. One thing in particular that I had to do was pee into a plastic thermos. The thermos was much like something you would take on a long hike through the mountains. It had a lid and measurements on the side for judging just how much urine I was producing on a daily basis. I heard a rumor that there was actually a thermos with a compass and Swiss army knife combo. I don't think that there were any that had a sippy straw, but why would there be? Given the right time of day, you could come into my hospital room, and find what looked to be a tall plastic container filled with a frothy, dark, delicious looking ale sitting at my bed side. I can guarantee that the contents did not contain hops.

Now when you are 14 and your friends are coming to visit, you can make jokes about a pee thermos all day long. But when it is a 14-year-old girl you know from school, or a friend of your mother's that you have never met before, a piping hot thermos of urine sitting on the table next to your bed is not something you flaunt or want people to notice. Often I would lay in bed and think, "What should I do with this thermos? Should I hide it under the sheets in bed with me? Should I just set it on the floor? What if I drop it? What if there is a leak? Will my bed smell like a toilet?" These are serious things to consider. When you lay in a hospital bed all day long there isn't much to do except watch TV and drink Coke. So filling the pee thermos was a fairly common occurrence. In all fairness to the nurses, they emptied the thermos on a regular basis. But inevitably, right after I finished drinking what seemed to be a gallon of orange juice and filling my thermos right to the top, a high ranking city official or the most beautiful girl I had ever seen would come knocking at my door.

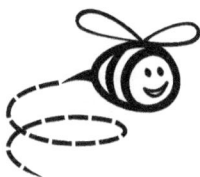

Chapter 3

A Discussion on Vomit

WHEN YOU ARE on chemotherapy, there aren't many times during the day when you feel like eating. There were times when I was in the hospital where I went days without eating so much as a cracker. I would often go so long without eating that I couldn't tell if the pain in my stomach was nausea or hunger. In the place of food, the hospital kept a running IV that looked like a giant bag of yellow Gatorade. It was basically just a solution to give me enough nutrients to keep from starving to death. But my doctors always encouraged me to eat anything I could, whenever I could. My gastro-enterologist would come in daily and ask me what I had eaten. Usually I would say nothing, but every now again I would mention some little morsel that I had had a craving for earlier that day.

I have never been pregnant, mainly because I am male, but I have heard that pregnant women often get strange cravings. I think people with cancer can relate. At night as I was in laying my bed, I would see commercials for food. Most of those commercials would just turn my stomach, but every now and then a commercial would catch my eye, and I would look to my mom or dad and say, "I have to have a Caesar salad right now!!" One night I was watching the movie *Weekend at Bernie's*, and the two main characters were eating foot long hot dogs, so of course I wanted foot long hot dog. My parents were so eager to have me eat anything, that they would go anywhere to get me anything at the drop of a hat. So if Caesar salad or a foot long hot dog is what I wanted, that is what I got. Upon returning with the Caesar salad however, my cravings would often change. Now I want pickles and ice cream! But I felt that since they went to the trouble to get the food, I should at least try eating a little bit of it.

When I was in the middle of my chemotherapy treatment, it was rare that I would eat anything and not vomit right after. Caesar salad, in my opinion, is a delicious food item; however, vomiting Caesar salad is not quite as delicious. It looks like collard greens or something Popeye would eat so he would stay strong to the finish. In the hospital if you want to vomit, and cannot get out of the bed on your own, you have two options: you can throw up all over yourself, or you can throw up into the giant plastic bucket that sits next to your bed. You may think that this is a no-brainer, but if you have thrown up enough times into this plastic bucket, it ALWAYS smells like vomit no matter how much or how well you wash it. It is like trying to throw up into a toilet that someone had just used but had not flushed. This may seem disgusting, and that's because it is! The bucket always smells like vomit!

I figured out eventually that I could get new buckets periodically, but after 3-5 vomit sessions it was back to the same old stench. So my favorite bucket coupled with freshly chewed Caesar salad, or perhaps a tuna sandwich with little celery bits, or maybe some spaghetti with meat sauce, resulted in one of my least favorite things to do, and that was vomit. I don't think there are too many people out there who ENJOY vomiting. But when you are in the hospital everything is scheduled. On Mondays I would have a certain chemo, at 12:00pm I would have blood work, I would get a bath every other day (more on that later). I knew when to expect these things. I had a sense of control. You have no control over when you throw up. There is no schedule. For a period of time, the only way I could control my vomiting was to not eat. I knew this wasn't healthy, so I would try and eat whatever sounded good whenever I could. In retrospect, when you don't eat for days, and then the first thing you put into your body is a Chalupa from Taco Bell, it probably makes sense that it would not sit well and you would have to throw up. As I weaned off my chemotherapy, I began throwing up less and less. I started to eat more and more, and eventually things got back to normal. After I was released from the hospital we kept a brand new plastic bucket next to my bed when I was on outpatient chemo therapy regiments for just-in-case moments. I don't know where that bucket is now. I know that I never used it, but I can still smell the plastic.

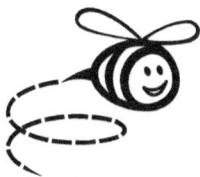

Chapter 4

Catheters and Sex Tapes

IN MEDICINE THERE are many uses of a catheter. The catheter that was used for me was a long, thin plastic tube inserted into my penis used to drain urine from my bladder. If there is a Heaven and there is a Hell, and these places were catered and specific to each individual based on their likes and dislikes, my specific Hell will involve a hospital bed, catheters, and a harem of hot nurses. Now for some of you readers, you may be thinking, wait a minute, this is my Heaven! But you wouldn't really think this if you have ever really experienced a catheter. When I was in the hospital, there were a few times where I had the privilege of experiencing a long plastic tube shoved down my urethra. This experience is not pleasant in any way. I don't know this for sure, but I think if you were to put a catheter under a microscope it would look similar to barbed wire or maybe a pipe cleaner. I am positive that there are tiny barbs along the tube. That coupled with the fact that all catheters seem to be approximately six feet in length makes it a sickening experience. The six feet may be an exaggeration but it sure does seem that long when a nurse is forcing a ball of fire into your genitals. I would rather a have poisoned dart shot into my crotch, because at least that would be quicker than a long tube made out of sandpaper.

Now to the harem of hot nurses! I have heard that it is a common male fantasy to be laid out in a hospital bed and have an extremely attractive nurse come into the room and she and the patient have a passionate night right there in the bed. I can tell you first hand that this NEVER happens. Most people who are in a hospital are there because they are sick, injured, and for the most part completely incapable of performing any illicit activity of any kind. When was the last time you looked at someone with pneumonia, or someone who just had a cardiac arrest, or in my case someone with leukemia, and thought, "I have to have sex with them right now!"? It doesn't happen. I was 14 when I was in the hospital, and a 14-year boy is in his prime when it comes to hormones. I know most of the nurses found me irresistible sexually.

With my patchy bald head from the chemotherapy, a 120-pound body from the lack of food, skin covered in acne due to steroid use, and open wounds from the tubes and procedures, my body pretty much sums up why a smoking hot nurse would want me. I took enough drugs on a day-to-day basis to kill a horse. But I was sure that a thirty-something nurse would see my vomit encrusted body and then want to commit statutory rape.

So my personal Hell would involve one of my doctors sneaking into my room late at night. He would quietly set up a tripod in the corner of my hospital room. He would place a camera on top of the tripod and frame the shot right on me sleeping soundly in my bed. He would be the sleazy doctor director of my own personal sex tape, in which I would be the star! He would cue the scene and it would go as follows:

SCENE: *Scott lies in bed and the lights are off in the room. The camera is in night vision mode. Slowly the door to his room opens, letting the light from the hall creep in next to the bed. A very attractive nurse sneaks into the room. She is dressed in a white nursing outfit that accentuates her curves. She quietly walks over to Scott in his bed. She softly strokes her hand across his acne-covered body. She runs her long luscious fingers through his patchy hair, and accidentally pulls out a clump of blonde strands. Scott awakens from his sleep. He sees the nurse before him and feels her hand moving slowly down towards his groin. At this moment Scott realizes his wildest dreams are about to come true. This nurse is going to turn him from a boy to a man. Scott looks at the nurse as her one hand approaches his groin and the other hand approaches her chest. Scott notices the nurse's hand close to her chest and sees that she is now reaching into a pocket on her nurse's uniform. Scott's pleasure quickly turns into horror as he realizes that her pocket contains a catheter! Scott looks over at his bedside clock. The clock reads 3:30am. Scott realizes that this isn't a sex tape, it is just time for his bladder to be drained! What was Scott's first and only sex tape has now become his nightly horror movie! The doctor and the nurse laugh maniacally as the door to the hospital room closes shut, covering the room in darkness, leaving only the sounds of Scott whimpering as the nurse slowly slides the barbed plastic tube into Scott's tiny pee hole.* END SCENE.

I think this movie is screaming to be made!

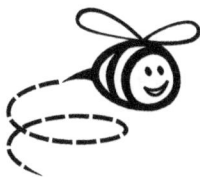

Chapter 5

It's Only a Little Toe

FAMILIES OFTEN FIND camaraderie amongst each other when their loved ones are in the hospital. I was in a children's hospital and there were a number of kids in the hospital for reasons that ran the gamut of afflictions. There were kids that were in for cancer, car accidents, heat strokes, and head injuries. Everything you can imagine. But regardless of why a child is in a hospital, the common bond that links them is that they are all there. Parents realize this quickly and stories are traded similarly to what I would imagine it would be like to be in prison. One mother will ask, "What are you guys in for?" A father may ask, "Any word on when you guys may get out of here?" These conversations help the parents cope, pass the time, and just find support from each other. Even though their kid may not have the exact same ailment, these parents have a better understanding of what they are going through than, say, a neighbor or co-worker.

There was a 2-3 week period when I was in the hospital where I was admitted into the intensive care unit. I had responded well to chemotherapy, but I may have responded a little too well, and I was left with a much depleted immune system. This left me open to infection, and a very serious infection is what I got. I developed a blood infection from bacteria called pseudomonas, and I also got pneumonia. I was on a large amount of medication, a respirator to help me breath, and I was kept heavily sedated. This 2-3 week period was a fog and I don't remember much of what took place during this time.

The initial night I was admitted to the ICU my parents were told that it was possible I may not live through the night. They had my father fill out organ donor papers just in case, which for me would be harder than actually hearing news that your son may die. It is funny that I don't really remember anything from that two to three week period of time, but I guess I am supposed to feel lucky or blessed or something that I survived. I guess I feel that way, but I was so detached from the experience that I don't really feel any way about it. I liken it to a story someone's mother may tell to their son or daughter when they are teenagers about something they did when they were a baby. "Oh when you were a baby you used to lie on the floor and eat bugs!" Well great!! How does that matter now? That is not to say I am not grateful that I am here today writing about it, but the bottom line is I survived the serious infection and now everyone was telling me how lucky and strong I am. But truth be told, I don't really know that I did anything but lay in a bed unconscious and have people pump me full of medication. I think the news that I was going to survive was more significant to my parents than to me.

The news was not all good, though. I had laid in bed for such a long time with little to no movement that my legs had atrophied and I had developed a condition called foot drop, where you aren't able lift your feet on your own to walk. The doctors had gotten my infection under control and it was clear that I wasn't going to die after all, but now they were telling my parents that I might only be able to walk with the help of leg braces and a cane. It was very unlikely that I would ever be able to run or play sports again. This was hard for me to accept, but I guess if the alternative choice is death, you can learn to live without badminton.

Once my stint in ICU ended, I was sent to the rehabilitation floor of the hospital. This is the place where you learn how to walk again and exercise and do all of the things that most of us take for granted every day. This was actually the hardest part for me both physically and mentally during my four-month stay in the hospital. When you lie in a bed for almost a month without moving like I did in ICU, it is amazing how completely inept you become at something so simple as standing up! The first few days I was on the rehab floor the physical therapists would strap me to something called a tilt table. The table laid flat and they would place me on the table, strap me down, and then it would tilt upright so that I was "standing" for roughly 20-30 minutes at a time. Afterwards they would lay the table flat again, and I felt as though I had just run a 10k race. It completely drained me of all of my energy. Just twenty minutes standing upright!

The whole learning-to-walk process was mentally draining as well. When my health improved I could notice a difference almost immediately. With physical therapy, though, the improvements are very slow. You can go a week or more without really noticing any change. Frustration set in, and I often became discouraged. But my dad was a bit of a drill sergeant when it came to my physical therapy. In looking back, he was exactly what I needed him to be. Taking a day off or not doing my exercises was not an option when he was around. He made sure that I always kept going and that I was always doing what I was supposed to do. Sure enough, I started to showed improvement. I started to walk again on my own, and I even started to show signs that I may get to run again and play sports with continued hard work.

While I was in ICU my mother met a comrade of sorts whose daughter was admitted for a variety of reasons. To be honest I don't even remember the exact reason why this little girl was in the hospital but the reason I do remember her is because her path was very similar to mine in the sense that when she was first admitted the prognosis of her surviving was not good. But she survived. The doctors told this girl's mother that the circulation in her daughter's legs wasn't very good and they thought they would have to amputate one or both of her legs. Hearing this news was hard to take but again with the alternative being death, amputated legs seemed like the lesser of two evils. The doctors were actually able to save both of her legs, and when it was all said and done, the only thing the little girl lost was her baby toe.

It is so funny how if you walked up to a random person on the street and asked them how they would feel about a doctor amputating their baby toe right then and there, they would probably be strongly against it. They would probably do a lot of things to keep that baby toe. But when you are in the hospital and dealing with one horrible thing after the other, you start to look at silver linings. My mother met a woman whose little girl survived a near-death experience, and her fee was only a baby toe. In the grand scheme of things it doesn't really seem like that much to pay. We can learn to live with and live without things when the alternative is something much worse. For me, I had survived, but the consequence was probably not being able to walk or run or doing any physical activity ever again. But it actually turned out I was able to walk without the help of braces or canes. I was able to learn to run again and I even made the varsity soccer team two years after I was released from the hospital. I remember very vividly running out onto the field for the first time. This was the first real soccer game I had played in about three years. I didn't play very well. In fact, I think my coach pulled me out of the game after about 10 minutes. But that was still way easier than that damn tilt table. Silver linings, right?

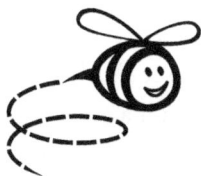

Chapter 6

The Keychain

BEING IN A hospital for an extended period of time can render one a bit of frustration to say the least. Depending on what ails you, you can have what seems like an endless amount of doctors, nurses, and hospital orderlies coming in an out of your room at every hour of the day. It is hard to get mad at them. I mean they are just doing to their job and their best I suppose to make sure that you get better and get out of the hospital as quickly as possible. But again, it is still hard not to get frustrated from time to time. There was a period where I had cancer doctors, heart and lungs doctors, stomach doctors, skin doctors, and they all would come in at different times (usually when I had just finally fallen asleep) to poke and prod different parts of my body. My favorite is when my IV drip would run out at 3am and the machine on the pole would start to beep until the nurse came in to change the bag and reset the unit. A hospital is really the last place you should go if you want a good night's sleep.

After a few weeks of being sick and being sleep-de-prived in a hospital, I started to get a little annoyed at a lot of different things. Luckily a small piece of plastic saved me from having multiple nervous breakdowns at the age of fifteen. This little plastic keychain was a small black box that had the usual silver key ring attached to the end. But why would this save my mental state you ask? Well, it was because of what the small black box could do! On one side of the box was a little speaker, and on the other side of the box were three small buttons. Pressing each of the three buttons produced a small voice that sounded like one of the three chipmunks. And each chipmunk said something different out of the little speaker on the other side. The phrases went as follows:

1. FUCK YOU!
2. FUCKING JERK
3. SON OF A BITCH

Now these three sayings are pretty offensive, but a fifteen year old hearing a chipmunk say any of these is wildly hilarious, and most of them could fit any situation of anger or frustration that I was feeling. If a doctor came in my room and told me that they were going to run a series of tests on me early in the morning, I would wait for the doctor to leave the room and I would lay in my bed with my keychain and proceed to press all three buttons over and over and over again until I laughed or at least felt a little better. Maybe I had a nurse or a nurse tech that wasn't so friendly or nice when they came into my room. I would wait for them to leave and then I would have the chipmunks tell them how I really felt. The funny thing is that over the months nurses and doctors would see the keychain on my bedside table and ask me about it, and almost all of them when hearing the phrases found it funny themselves. It became so accepted that I had this keychain, that my mom actually got me a piece of sticky Velcro so that I could attach it to the rail guard on my hospital bed. If my friends came to visit me in the hospital, the keychain was right there and hours were spent creating scenarios where the keychain could be used.

My stomach doctor would like to come in my room to do my check up at around seven in the morning when I was still sleeping every single day. Towards the end of my stay at the hospital, after he would do his check up, he would reach over to the little black keychain stuck to my rail guard and push a button as if to say, "Sorry I came in to bug you while you were sleeping, I am a f**king jerk!" That keychain is pretty inappropriate in a lot of situations. I could have never brought it to school. It wouldn't have been a very good way to start off an important business meeting, and it wouldn't be a very good icebreaker for a first date. But somehow in the hospital it was just accepted. My doctors, my nurses, and my parents all sort of just knew being a kid in a hospital is hard. It is hard to stay positive, it is hard not to get angry, and it is hard to not get frustrated. That keychain allowed some chipmunks to express some of my feelings for me. It allowed me to blow off some steam when I needed to.

When I was released from the hospital I took the keychain home with me and eventually the battery died, and the need for it sort of died with it. The keychain is long gone by now but it was just as important to me as anything else that I had while I was in the hospital. I think if someone is admitted into a hospital no matter their age or their reason for being there, they should be given a hospital hospitality package. It should be filled with things like an mp3 player, a subscription to netflix, and most importantly a little black keychain with some type of little rodent screaming expletives at the top of their little rodent lungs.

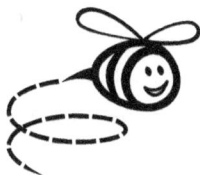

Chapter 7

Have You Seen My Weiner?

WHEN I WAS growing up, I was always a very guarded little boy. I was my mom and dad's first born and I think my parents were a little over protective when I was young, which in turn caused me to be a little over dramatic. I don't mean to say that my parents were over bearing or protective in a bad way. They just treated me like a first-born. When I spilled something they were right there to clean it up. If my shirt got dirty they would change it right away. When my little brother was born they had already been through it and kind of knew what to expect. So needless to say when my brother and I ate at the table, I ate about as neatly as a five year old could eat, while my brother was covered in peanut butter.

I have always said I have had a 401k since I was eight. This continued throughout my time in elementary school, as well. My books always had to fit a certain way in my desk, and I always had to have all of my stuff in my pencil box arranged in a certain way. When I was in elementary school we had P.E., but you didn't really have to dress out for it. You could wear whatever clothes you had on, and basically you could just run around a field for about a half hour. But when I entered the seventh grade as my first year of middle school, I learned that I would have to "dress out" for gym. This meant change from jeans or pants into running shorts. I was going to have to change clothes in front of other boys in a locker room in order to make good grades in class.

Now this may not seem like a big deal to a lot of people, but this literally kept my thirteen-year-old mind wide awake at night. I quickly learned that I could wear my gym shorts underneath my jeans to school. That way when I got into the locker room, all I would have to do is take my jeans off and viola, I was dressed out for gym. My dad would tell me stories that they would actually have to shower after gym when he was a kid and that was just too much for me to even think about. When I was at home and alone I would have showered with clothes on if I could have for fear that someone may walk in on me.

The only reason I didn't is because I would have had to explain why all of my clothes were wet to my mother. If I had to shower at school I would have worn a wet suit to gym so I would not have to take my clothes off in front of other people.

Everything I just wrote about is completely true but something happened to me the summer I turned fifteen. I got cancer. Being in a hospital will do more to squash any inhibition or modesty that you have quicker than you can say gym shorts. When all of those doctors and nurses mentioned in previous chapters come into your room during the day or in the night, they want to make sure everything is ok and I do mean everything. Being a male in the hospital, it was a regular thing for my doctors to make sure that the cancer had not spread to different areas of my body. One big place was my brain and spinal fluid, but they also wanted to check my glands and genitals. Over the course of a few months I became comfortable enough to be able to drop my pants for a few select doctors so they could give me a good once over and then that was that, no big deal. But after my stay in ICU I had a hard time standing and walking. Heading over to a bathtub for a shower all of a sudden became very hard work. Believe it or not, even though I was just lying around in a bed all day doing absolutely nothing, a couple of days without a bath left me smelling like my pee thermos. Baths became necessary and the hospital had an ingenious way of bathing me without me ever taking a step.

Down in the basement of the hospital there was this giant metal whirlpool that they could fill with piping hot water. Next to the whirlpool was a giant contraption that looked like a crane that had a flat base connected to a chain, and at the end of the chain was a piece of green canvas that looked a little bit like a hammock. Every other day I was helped into my wheel chair, and I was taken to the basement where the giant metal whirlpool contained thousands of gallons of scalding hot water. Once I got to the basement I had to take off all of my clothes and a pack of about five hospital employees, most of whom I had never met, lifted my pale naked body onto the piece of green canvas connected to the crane like contraption. After this I was lifted by the chain and swung wildly across the room, still naked, dangling over the boiling whirlpool. Every time I had a bath I felt like some sort of livestock being placed into holding pen right before that weight slams them in the back of the head killing them instantly. That would have been less humiliating than the naked teenager on a crane baths that I had.

After I was lowered into the fiery molten lava, I would get to wash myself, while every single person who had a shift in the hospital at that time had decided it was time to check out this mysterious whirlpool that they had heard so much about. I have to say that I love washing my penis underwater while a parade of janitors, nurses, and cafeteria workers came through the whirlpool room one after the other. I am almost positive that my crotch became the most watched program on the closed circuit channel on the hospital television. By the end of my stay in the hospital I was willing to show my junk to anybody and everybody, whether they asked to see it or not. My modesty pretty much went out of the window while I was there. After I got out of the hospital, it didn't take me long to sort of get back to my old ways. When I joined the soccer team in high school a couple of years after I was sick, I was still a little guarded about changing my clothes in front of my teammates, but I was definitely a little less shy than I was before. I will say that if I am ever admitted back into a hospital for whatever reason, the first question I am asking is whether or not they have a whirlpool.

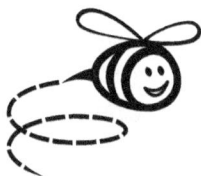

Chapter 8

It's a Lot Like a Bee Sting

I WAS DIAGNOSED WITH leukemia and admitted to a hospital on a Friday night. Obviously, I
was scared, but mostly because I had no idea what
to expect in the coming weeks and, as it turned out,
months. Since I was diagnosed on a Friday, I was told
that I wouldn't start my chemotherapy regiment until
that following Monday. Every chemo regiment is special for every patient depending on things like how long
the person has had cancer before starting treatment, how
severe the cancer actually is, and how much it has spread.
The two main places in my body that my doctors needed
to check were my spinal fluid and my bone marrow. The
spinal fluid was important because if the cancer spread
there it would have been very hard to get out. My doctors

wanted to check my bone marrow because that was what was producing these bad white blood cells in my body. I was told they were going to check both of these things over the weekend so that they would know how to proceed with my treatment plan for Monday.

Now the procedures for both of these things involve very large needles and a pretty good amount of pain. To check my spinal fluid they were going to do a lumbar puncture, sometimes called a spinal tap. I was told that this involved me curling up into a ball on a table so that spine was poking out. Then my doctor took a needle that was about a foot long and inserted it into one of the vertebrae in my lower back. The end of the needle had a nozzle that connected to a little glass vile, which allowed my spinal fluid to drip out into the vile. If the fluid was clear like water, everything was good. However, if the fluid was cloudy or milky looking, then that meant trouble. Luckily, my spinal fluid was always crystal clear.

They said that the procedure was a little painful but that it was quick. But the bone marrow was the one that most kids had a problem with. Now to me, a good doctor is someone who gives the facts and is honest and up front, but at the same time reassuring and comforting. When a doctor says something is going to hurt that means it is going to hurt like hell. The bone marrow check is similar in nature to the spinal tap, but for this one I was told I was going to lay flat, stomach down on a table and they would take another foot long needle into my hip bone. The needle was attached to a syringe and they were going to draw some bone marrow out of my pelvis. This big difference between the two procedures actually had nothing to do with needles or doctors, but with my own body. The hipbone is quite a bone! It is thick, sturdy, and is meant to withstand some wear and tear. In order to puncture the hipbone, which was what they were going to do, this was going to require some serious hardware. Needless-to-say, I started to really freak out.

That Friday night I laid in my bed thinking only of the two procedures that I would have the next morning and all I could picture was my doctor coming out of a back room with a needle the size one of the those swords they use in fencing tournaments telling me to relax because this was going to be the worst pain I had ever felt in my life. My mom and my dad were being pretty good parents telling me it was going to be fine and over before I knew it, but to be honest, it really wasn't assuaging any bad feelings I was having.

Later on that night, though, something odd happened. I was watching TV...just trying to relax. The door to my hospital room was ajar and I heard a very small little knock. Standing there was a little boy with no hair and who couldn't have been older than 7 or 8. He was wearing a hospital gown like you always see in the movies and he was wheeling his IV pole around with him. I said hello to him and we started talking. I found out that he was a couple of rooms down from me and he also had leukemia. He had been in and out of the hospital for a little over a month. I don't know how he found out it was my first night. Maybe a nurse told him to come down and talk to me, maybe my parents told the little boy's parents, who knows. That conversation with that little boy was one of the most significant moments I had in the hospital and it happened the very first night.

During our conversation the little boy asked me when I was scheduled to have my spinal tap and bone marrow check. I told him that I was scheduled for both in the morning. The boy told me that he had already had more than one of each and he described to me that each procedure was "a lot like a bee sting." A bee sting? That's it? Right then and there I had a moment of clarity. A seven year old boy had been able to deal with more than one spinal tap and more than one bone marrow check, and the only reaction that it got from him was that it was like a bee sting. I heard this and knew that I had to suck it up. This is what I had to do. If I wanted to live, I didn't have another choice. This is not to say I never got frustrated or discouraged but whenever I did I remembered that boy and I just kept thinking to myself that it was going to be a lot like a bee sting. My parents were always supportive and encouraging, and I really think I had one of the best doctors you could have, but nothing they said gave me as much courage and confidence as that little boy. Seeing him and seeing that he was going through treatment and succeeding gave me hope the very first night I was in the hospital. It completely changed my outlook on the way things were going to go. I wish every cancer patient, on his or her first or second day of treatment, could have the opportunity to talk with a survivor or at least someone who is succeeding with treatment. I never saw that little boy after that first weekend. I don't even remember his name. I like to think he has grown up and is doing well. I was inspired to write this book because of him.

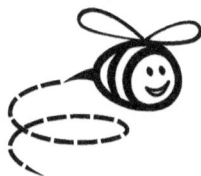

Chapter 9

Sweet Dreams

DURING MY TREATMENT I was literally on drugs. I mean I wasn't doing heroin or crack, but I was on stuff that made me hallucinate like I was in the front row at Woodstock. When I would take naps during the day, I would have wild, vivid dreams that I often had a hard time telling the difference between these dreams and reality. There were two recurring dreams in particular that were especially kooky. The first had an international feel. The dream would span the entire day and go into the evening. During the day I was out on an African safari. I lived in a village with my dad. Our house was made out of a giant elephant skeleton. The giant rib cage of the elephant skeleton was the shell of the house. I would spend all day lying underneath the

39

elephant rib cage trying to stay out of the hot sun. My dad would stay there with me for the day and prepare me for my daily beating.

I know this probably sounds more like a nightmare, but every time I had this dream at one point in the late afternoon a man would drive in to our village and up to our elephant rib cage. He would get off his bike and place his front wheel right on my chest. He would then grip the handlebar and crank the throttle over and over again spinning the front tire on my chest. In real life this would probably kill someone, but in my dream it was more like someone just slapping me over and over in the chest. It was painful, but not lethal. After about a half hour spinning that tire on my chest, the motorcycle man would leave and the sun would set.

At this point my dream would shift locations. I would leave the heat of the African safari and jet to the city life of Tokyo, Japan. This part of the dream took place in the penthouse of the fanciest hotel in all of Tokyo. My father was no longer in the dream, but my aunt and uncle replaced him. They were throwing a champagne party at the top of this hotel. There wasn't anyone else in the dream that I knew or recognized but the strangest part of this dream was that all of the champagne was being served by large silverback gorillas wearing tuxedos. I remember being very thirsty in this part of the dream, but every time I would approach a gorilla with a tray they would turn and go the other way. Nothing else really happened in the dream, but I remember it being so real that one afternoon I woke up from a drug induced dream and asked my dad where the gorillas were. He would just laugh because he knew I had just been tripping on some sort of cocktail the nurses had given me earlier that day.

The second dream always involved my mother. In the dream, she worked in the hospital as a clown. She would push around a giant white cart on wheels that had six big white tubs filled with different flavors of sherbet. To this day I have no idea if my mom actually did this at one point or if it was all in my head. But if it wasn't real it was the most lifelike dream I had ever had. My clown mother had little bowls and spoons on top of her cart and she would go from room to room and give every sick little kid a bowl of sherbet. As she walked down the hall, all of the nurses would fight each other for access to the sherbet. What kind of nurses steal sherbet from sick children? Evil nurses in crazy dreams. This dream didn't have all of the flare and international flavor as the other one, but it wasn't any less crazy. Two years after I got out of the hospital, I went to a party that was thrown by a kid in my 11th grade science class. Like an after school special, another

41

kid approached me at the party and offered me drugs. I told him no thanks, I hadn't done drugs in two years and I was trying to keep the gorillas out of my head.

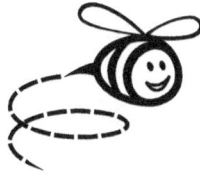

Chapter 10

Everything Happens for a Reason

SPIRITUALITY IS A big part of many people's lives, regardless of whether or not they have a life threatening disease. There were many families that I met while in the hospital where their faith was very important. There was a chapel in the children's hospital where families could go on Sunday for church service or just go to pray or think or whatever it was that they needed to do. This chapter is in no way about me trying to convert any reader to a specific faith or religion. But I think faith and belief is a central theme to one's journey through disease and struggle. I think it is almost impossible to be told that you have a disease that may result in death, and not question your existence and your reason for being. My parents, I think, also struggled with these ideas. I think it is in our nature to want to justify everything that happens in the world especially when it is something that is bad. Murderers always need motives, death always needs a cause, and my family and I were trying to justify disease. My parents and some of my relatives always told me that everything happens for a reason. That notion really stuck with me for a long time.

The last month I was in the hospital, and the years following, I was an angry person. I walked around every day looking for arguments and looking for reasons to fly off the handle. When I was in college I got in trouble for leaving a curse filled tirade on the voice mail of the registrar's office because they didn't open theirs doors before 9am during the week of registration and I couldn't do registration online. So I called them up and told them what I thought of them. That call got me in a little bit of trouble with the school, but I learned from it. When I was a teenager I tried to choke my brother once on our couch but I don't even remember why. For a while I almost took pride in the fact that I had a short temper. It was something that defined who I was, but over the years I realized that losing my temper never really resulted in anything positive. I usually got into trouble or hurt someone I cared about.

The older I got, the less having a short temper seemed like a good thing to have. So rather than take pride in my temper I tried to think about reasons why I felt this way. What had made me so angry? I think it really started when my parents were divorced, but I think it was exacerbated when I got sick a couple years later. I realized after thinking a lot about it that it would only be natural to have anger issues over these things. I think all emotions are healthy, including anger, if they are handled in productive ways, and I definitely was not handling my anger productively. I knew lots of kids whose parents were divorced, and through my experience I met a lot of kids who also had cancer, but none of them were having emotional breakdowns when they went to the movies and it was sold out. So again I tried to think about what was making my anger so intense. I came to the realization that one little phrase was doing it. One little sentence was making me fight something or someone every day: Everything happens for a reason. The justification that I had heard countless times from family, friends, and even doctors was at the heart of my anger.

For me, when I heard everything happens for a reason, I automatically thought to the future. I thought that the reason I had cancer would show itself somewhere down the road. That somehow something would eventually happen in my life and it would give me clarity on why I had cancer. I would have that "aha" moment where I would finally say, "This is it! Now I know why I had cancer! This is the reason!" The problem is you can go every day expecting something to happen, waiting for that monumental event to take place. What if that event doesn't show itself until I am sixty or older? That is a long time to wait for justification. I guess one could argue that maybe it doesn't have to be one giant event but a series of small events that when all added together will lead to that "aha" moment. I suppose that is true too, but how small are these events? Will I even notice that they happen? What if they initially seem so insignificant that I miss most of them and then never get my justification?

I began to spend more and more time thinking about this and then something else occurred to me. I always spun the phrase "everything happens for a reason" to the future, but the more I thought about it I started to think about the past. I started to think that if everything happens for a reason, then I must have done something to be selected to have cancer. This revelation I decided was the heart of my problem. What could I have done in the first fourteen years of my life that warranted leukemia? Why was I chosen? When I thought about this I got really angry. I felt anger like I had never felt before. I am not a perfect person, but I couldn't think of one thing that I had done in my life that would have resulted in the grand prize of cancer. This little phrase, "everything happens for a reason," can cause a person to go crazy thinking about what they did in the past and what was to come in the future.

I struggled with it every day for a long time, and one day I had a thought: What if everything *doesn't* happen for a reason? When people get a sinus infection, is there a big plan or reason for it or did they just get a cold? Why should it be any different for someone with cancer? Maybe I just got sick. Maybe there was no reason or plan or destiny. Was I still angry I got cancer and that I spent almost a year of my life in the hospital? Of course! But taking out all of the reasoning and justification lifted a weight off my shoulders that allowed me to deal with it instead of struggling with what I had done in the past and what was going to happen in the future. I have mellowed out a bit over the past few years. There have still been a few occasions where I have lost my temper easier than I should have. Every few months I will still think about being sick and old feelings will start to come back, but I think that is only natural. My experience with cancer will obviously stay with me forever. But those times are fewer and far between. Part of it is being 28 years old instead of 18 years old. I like to think I am more mature, and I have learned over the years how to take my anger and be less reactive and more proactive. In all fairness to me, though, whenever I get angry lately there is always a really good reason!

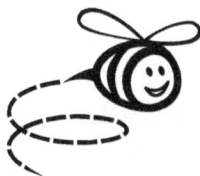

Chapter 11

And All I Got Was
This Lousy T-Shirt

I WAS DIAGNOSED WITH leukemia in March of 1995 and released from the hospital in August that same year. That was a long five months, but my treatment didn't end in August. I actually was on a small dosage of chemotherapy for the next five years. I had spinal taps every three months and monthly appointments every three to four weeks. It was a long journey. A very long journey. I was in remission from cancer, I was back in school, and my hair had even started to grow back. For all intents and purposes I was a normal kid, but leukemia still consumed almost every day of my life for five straight years. There was rarely a day where I didn't think about cancer, talk about cancer, or experience it in the form of doctors or hospitals. It sat like a weight on my shoulders. It was a part of me but sometimes I kept certain things to myself, because I didn't want to be the guy who just talks about his cancer all of the time. So there were a lot of times where I kept emotions and ideas bottled. I am pretty sure that contributed to some of my anger and slight depression that I experienced after the fact. It was even difficult for me to go to celebratory events. There were always survivor rallies at water parks or banquets, but to me it was just another reminder of what I was dealing with everyday. On a side note, every one of these survivor rallies had hot dogs as a food option. I feel like there has been extensive research that hot dogs have carcinogens yet everywhere you turn people are serving cancer survivors hot dogs. What gives?

After I finished my treatment my grandmother would always try to get me to participate in Race for the Cure, or Relay for Life, or Camp Sunshine. All of these things are wonderful programs and I am not trying to belittle anything these organizations do. However, I think it is hard sometimes for people to understand that cancer dominated my everyday life for five straight years, and when I was told I was done with treatment and chemo and spinal taps, all I wanted to do was completely and totally distance myself from everything involved with cancer. I wasn't ready to just turn around and start doing Relay for Life and immerse myself in that again. That is not to say that this approach is for everyone. There are lots of people who find strength and encouragement and support with these events. That is the whole reason why they were created. But for me at the time, I wanted nothing to do with them.

The last official day of my treatment I went in to the doctor and he gave me one last physical and he and all the nurses were ready to send me on my way. But before I left they gave me a parting gift. It was a t-shirt that said, "Accept any challenge." My first thought was, "I had cancer and all I get is a goddamn t-shirt?" But actually I really didn't expect anything going into the doctor that day so after I thought about it, it turned out to be kind of a pleasant surprise. I still have that shirt and over the last couple of years, I have realized that enough time has passed and I have really started to participate in a lot of different activities. I have done a Relay for Life each of the last two years. I also run in 5k races around Atlanta that benefit skin and breast cancer. I even decided it would be a good idea to write a book. I guess you the reader will decide whether or not that was really a good idea.

I am not trying to impress by writing about these things but my point is that I don't think people who have had cancer should feel like they have to do anything or feel pressured to do anything they are not comfortable with. I think if people want to participate in breast cancer walks, or a teenager wants to go to Camp Sunshine because it will make them feel good and proud and supported, then I think that is great. But I also think that if there is a period of time where they want to leave it all behind, then that is what they should do, too. I have known many teenagers who have parents that make them do some of the aforementioned things. I always tell them that they were the ones who had cancer and not their parents, and they should do what makes them feel comfortable. Sometimes when we are young we don't always know how and when to speak up for ourselves. But speaking up for ourselves and saying what we feel is the only way we know we are still alive, and as long as we continue to do that, cancer will never win.

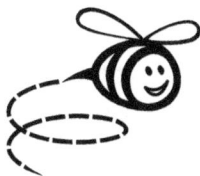

Chapter 12

Vive La France!

I AM WRITING THIS right now from my hotel in France. Well that is partially true. I was worried that my computer would be stolen or damaged while traveling, so I have decided to write the old fashioned way and that is with a pen and paper. I will transfer this to my computer when I get back. I will say this up front: This chapter is totally for me and not the reader. It was fourteen years ago that I went to France with my mom. The last day of that trip I woke up with half of my face paralyzed, and thus begun my stint with cancer. When I went to college, French turned out to be my minor so I have actually been to France two times since then. But both of those trips were with school groups and they had a much different vibe. They were very structured and had very rigid itineraries and I didn't really have time to re-flect on my previous trips. This voyage is special because I have traveled with my wife. In a lot of ways it is very similar to the trip I took with my mom. It is just the two of us, and we can kind of go and do whatever we want whenever we want.

Yesterday we went to the top of the Eiffel Tower. It was windy, cold, and rainy. Very similar to when I went to the top of the Eiffel Tower with my mom fourteen years ago. So why am I including all of this information in this book? Because there are things that go on in life that will make you think about those times when you were sick, or things that led up to when you were sick. There was a movie that came in out in the '90s called *The River Wild*. It starred Meryl Streep and Kevin Bacon, and it was a pretty good movie. I saw it for the first time about three weeks before I was diagnosed with leuke-mia. The night I watched it, I was at my dad's apartment and we had chicken patties for dinner. I spent the whole last half of that movie throwing up chicken patties into my dad's toilet and trashcan. From that night forward, I spent the next two months throwing up regardless of what I ate or drank. Whenever I see *The River Wild* on TV I think about that night. My friend once got really sick off of Philly cheesesteaks, and he can no longer eat

Philly cheesesteaks. I actually still like chicken patties. I couldn't eat them for a while, but my disdain for them has waned over the years, and I have grown to like them again. But I still think about that night.

There are songs that I hear on the radio that were popular that summer, and I immediately think about being on the rehab floor in the hospital learning how to walk again or riding an exercise bicycle. It is weird to me that none of these things are necessarily negative in my life. Sometimes there are things in life that we want to forget. Maybe a horrible date, or a verbal faux pas, but I have really tried to make an effort to hold onto some of the good memories of that whole experience. How could I possibly have good memories from spending five months in the hospital with cancer? There were moments, albeit short ones, that I actually remember as happy moments while I was there.

One afternoon I remember watching the movie *Dumb and Dumber* with my brother and friends in my hospital room. That is in my top five hardest laughs I have ever had in my life. Every morning before I would go into the rehab room to do my daily exercises and training, my dad and I would watch SportsCenter or read the sports section in the newspaper and complain about how our respective baseball teams were terrible. That was one of my favorite parts of the day. Whenever my mom was in my hospital room, I always felt less nervous or scared. There aren't always a ton of positive things you can take away from having cancer, but after sifting through all of those anger issues that I mentioned in Chapter 10, it is great to think about the few positive things that happened as a result of my illness.

So as I sit here on my bed in my hotel in Paris, I can think about that trip that my mom and I took in 1995. I try not to think about it as the trip where I got cancer. I think of it as just a great trip with my mom. I mean I don't think that the country of France gave me cancer, although I think there are people who would argue differently. Most of them have never been here though. I think it would be fun someday for my mom and me to go back to France together. Not to erase old memories, but to create new ones. Not to dwell on the past, but to think of the future. I look forward to that one day and getting all of the sweet souvenirs. Vive La France!

*Souvenir is the french verb for "to remember"...do you get it!?

www.ingramcontent.com/pod-product-compliance
Lightning Source LLC
Chambersburg PA
CBHW022131280326
41933CB00007B/641